ways
to fall
ASLEEP

100 hacks for when
you can't get to sleep

An Hachette UK Company
www.hachette.co.uk

First published in Great Britain in 2020 by
Pyramid, an imprint of Octopus Publishing
Group Ltd
Carmelite House, 50 Victoria
Embankment, London EC4Y 0DZ
www.octopusbooks.co.uk

ISBN 978-0-75373-403-2

A CIP catalogue record for this book is
available from the British Library

Printed and bound in China

10 9 8 7 6 5 4 3 2 1

Publisher: Lucy Pessell
Designer: Hannah Coughlin
Junior Editor: Sarah Kennedy
Editorial Assistant: Emily Martin

Production Controller: Grace O'Byrne

Picture acknowledgements
p.7 unsplash/Andy Holmes; p.9 Andrew
Easton
Freepik.com: cover and endpapers
designed by Freepik; brushstrokes designed
by rawpixel.com; p.72 designed by Freepik
iStock/Tetiana Lazunova: p.22, p.38,
p.120, p.121
Noun Project: pencil and brush icons
Daria Moskvina; p.14 b farias; p.18
Cantasia; p.24 Pawinee E.; p.30 Made
by Made; p.44 Fernando Affonso; p.49
Dara Ullrich; p.53 Shannon Dunlop; p.60
Alice Noir; p.61 Laymik; p.61 Oleksandr
Panasovskyi; p.70 BT Hai; p.74 Maxicons;
p.96 newstudiodesign; pp.110-110 Linseed
Studio

Introduction

Do you find yourself struggling to sleep at night, helplessly trying to clear your mind only to watch the hours slip by? You aren't alone. In our current hectic and non-stop world, drifting off isn't always easy. There are myriad distractions keeping us up at night: smartphones, street lighting, noisy neighbours, not to mention the stress and pressure of everyday modern life.

But fear not; here is the perfect collection of tips, tricks and activities to help you overcome your sleep problems. Work through them in any order you wish, whether it's a bit of colouring-in or list-making that you fancy, or just a few helpful pointers as to what might help you drift off for the night. Some are designed to relax you by helping you get your thoughts straight in your head. Others are just a bit of fun when you need a distraction late at night.

Make sure you're comfy. Sit back, relax and discover all the ways to fall asleep.

Wear an eye mask

It can often be hard to achieve total darkness in your bedroom at night, whether your flatmates or family members tend to leave lights on in hallways, or if light from streetlamps and passing cars gets in through your bedroom window. Wearing an eye mask can improve your sleep by blocking out all of that excess light, helping you to drift off into a deeper and better quality snooze.

Hug something

Did you know that hugging a pillow or blanket to sleep
can help reduce feelings of stress and anxiety? This
is because cuddling suppresses the effects of cortisol,
the stress hormone, making us feel calmer and more
relaxed. Try snuggling up to your favourite pillow or
blanket and see if you feel a little sleepier.

Labyrinth Meditation

Trace your finger over this night-sky labyrinth, following the path from one end to the other.

As you trace the curves, let your mind relax and empty of all distracting thoughts.

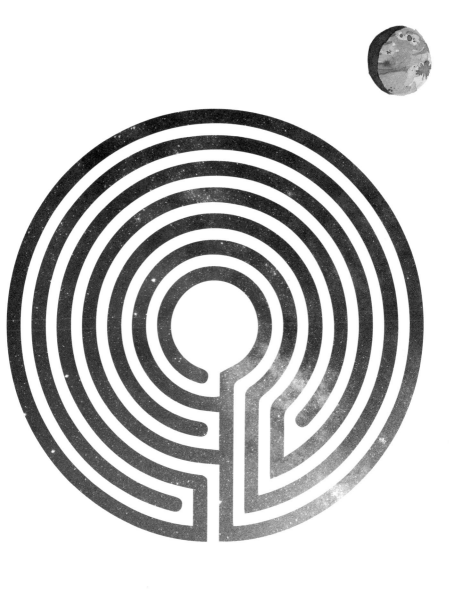

Dot-to-dot

Complete this stress-busting dot-to-dot to help clear your head. Watch the illustration slowly take form as you find a sense of satisfaction that will help clear your mind.

When you reach a hollow dot, lift your pen and return it to the page on the following number.

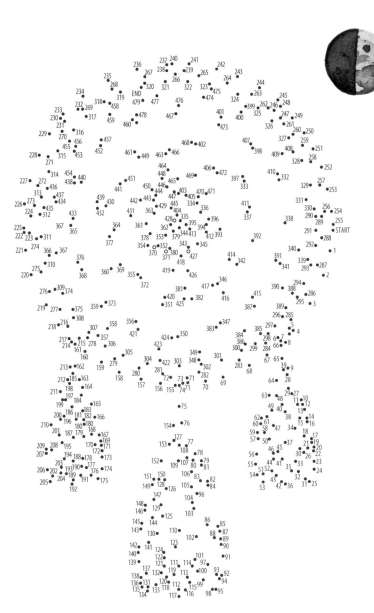

Turn off blue light

Blue light emitted from your smartphone, tablet or laptop screen is especially disruptive to your circadian rhythm, the natural process that controls your sleep–wake cycle. Make sure all of your devices are switched onto night mode for a better and more restful sleep.

Listen to white noise

When you're in a completely silent room, the odd creak of a floorboard or the tick of a clock can be really distracting. Try turning on some white noise to drown out all of those little sounds – there are plenty of apps available to download.

Face your fears

Use this space to write down any of your fears or worries, or anything that's stopping you from sleeping right now. Getting them down on paper and out of your head will help you feel calmer.

Be thankful

It's so easy to dwell on the bad parts of your day and to let negative thoughts build up in your head, stopping you from getting to sleep. Use this space to write down all the things to be thankful for. This will lift your mood and put your mind at rest.

....

....

....

....

....

....

....

....

Lower the temperature

The quality of your sleep may be improved by lowering the temperature of your bedroom. This is because your body's core temperature must fall slightly in order for the process of sleep to begin.

Aim to keep your bedroom between 15°C/60°F and 20°C/68°F for a better night's sleep.

Have a hot shower

This works in a similar way to the previous tip, and can be a faster way to lower your core body temperature. By stepping out of a hot shower and immediately into cooler surroundings, your body will transfer heat from its central core to areas such as your hands and feet, from which heat can be lost more easily. This in turn will lower your core temperature, readying your body for sleep.

Mandala colouring

A mandala is a sacred circle, a symbol of wholeness. They are usually circular and are always symmetrical, drawing your eye towards their central element.

Colouring intricate designs demands mental focus and concentration. This focus naturally causes you to suspend your mental chatter, achieving a kind of mindfulness that will leave you feeling calmer.

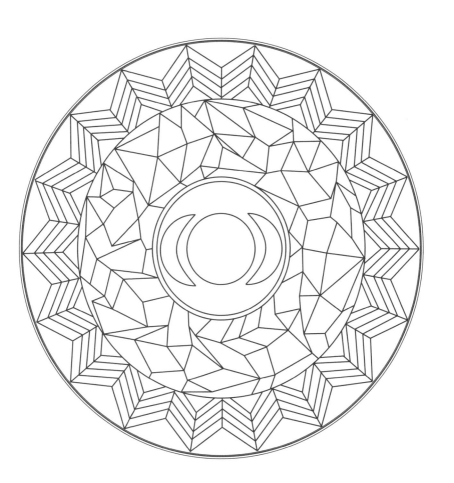

Read your favourite book

Try getting cosy with your favourite book or magazine, or whatever makes you feel relaxed and calm. Notice the comforting familiarity of the words as you read, and how they make you feel safe and at ease in your surroundings.

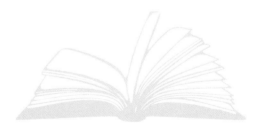

Wear earplugs

If you're a particularly light sleeper, and even the slightest sound can keep you from nodding off, try putting in some earplugs to achieve total silence at night.

Breathe

Complete this breathing exercise to help relax
your body and clear your mind.

You may find it helps to do this exercise regularly
before bed. Incorporate it into your night routine
and see if it helps you switch off.

You can do this exercise either sitting or lying down.

Making sure you are comfortable, completely relax your arms and legs.

Take a slow, deep breath in through your nose, letting the air fill your lungs and stomach as much as is comfortable.

Breathe all the way out again, continuing to keep your arms and legs relaxed. When you think there is no air left, try to breathe out just that little bit more so that you completely empty your lungs.

Repeat as many times as you wish, but three to five minutes should help you feel more relaxed.

Yoga

Yoga can help relax your mind and stretch out any parts of your body that may be feeling tense and tight after a long day.

The following pose is a quick and easy way to relieve any tension in your body.

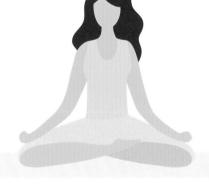

Viparita Karani (legs up the wall pose)

Find some open wall space. Start by sitting on the floor with the left side of your body up against the wall. As you breathe out, slowly lie down on your back and gently pivot yourself so that the backs of your legs are touching the wall, and your feet are facing upwards. Take as much time as you need to do this. You may find you have to shuffle around a bit to get into a comfortable position.

Don't worry if you can't get your bottom right up against the wall – just find the position that feels best.

Rest your arms at your sides, and hold the pose for five to ten minutes.

Shut down your devices

If you can't think of any good reason why you might need to keep your phone, tablet or laptop on overnight, turn it off! This'll help curb the temptation to have that quick look through your social media feeds. It'll also mean you aren't disturbed by any lights or notification sounds as you sleep.

If you really must keep your phone on, leave it on silent with the screen faced down.

Make a hot water bottle

You may have already read about the importance of lowering your body temperature and keeping the room cool, but a freezing cold environment isn't going to help either. If you're struggling to warm up at night, try getting extra cosy with a hot water bottle, and get rid of it once you feel warm enough. This will prevent your body from overheating.

Create a playlist

Listen to songs that make you feel relaxed and at ease. Try to avoid anything too upbeat or energizing. Why not explore some gentle jazz or classical music? Write down a list of your go-to songs so you don't forget them.

Stretch

Stretch out any parts of your body that are feeling particularly tight or tense at the end of the day.

Start at the top of your body, slowly stretching each body part as you move down towards your feet.

Sleep in total darkness

If you don't have an eye mask, try to achieve total darkness in your room by making sure your curtains are closed properly. Make sure any annoying lights in landings and hallways are switched off, too.

Total darkness will help increase your melatonin levels – the hormone that tells your body it's time for bed – and will also improve the quality of your sleep.

Get good pillow placement

Depending on which position you like to sleep in, arranging your pillow in different ways might help you get more comfortable:

If you sleep on your back, you may find that a small pillow underneath your knees will help support the natural curve of your back.

If you sleep on your side, try putting a pillow between your knees to reduce stress on your hips and lower back.

If you sleep on your front, a flat pillow underneath your pelvis may help to keep your spine aligned.

Drink chamomile tea

Chamomile tea contains lots of sleep-inducing antioxidants, and can help make you feel a little sleepier when it comes to bedtime.

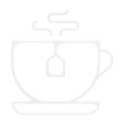

Make use of lavender

There are plenty of room and pillow sprays available that contain soothing scents, such as lavender, that can help you feel more relaxed at night. Lavender has long been known to help calm and comfort, and may help you nod off that bit quicker.

Massage your head

Giving yourself a head massage will relax your head and neck muscles, and can help to relieve any tension that has built up during the day.

The following instructions will show you how to massage your head for the best results.

Making sure you're comfortable, start by massaging your scalp with the pads of your fingers in a circular motion.

Putting pressure on the area at the base of your head and at the top of your neck can help to relieve built-up tension.

Pressure on either side of the upper nose, where your eyebrows start, can help to treat eye strain.

Don't get cold feet

Warming up your feet causes vasodilation – dilation of the blood vessels – which can send signals to your brain telling it that it's time for sleep.

Try wearing some fluffy socks to sleep, or put a hot water bottle at the foot of the bed for cosy feet as you drift off.

Listen to a podcast

There are lots of podcasts out there designed specifically for when you can't get to sleep. Have a browse online or on streaming services, and see what takes your fancy.

Make a to-do list

Making a to-do list for the next day can help put your mind at rest. By having a solid plan for the next day, you don't have to spend time worrying about what needs doing the night before. Use the space below to write down some key tasks you'd like to get done. Why not separate your list into daily, weekly and yearly to-dos.

Don't just lie there

If you're really struggling to sleep, and it's been over twenty minutes, try getting up and moving to a different room and doing something relaxing like reading a book or listening to gentle music. This way, your body won't associate any feelings of frustration and stress with being in bed.

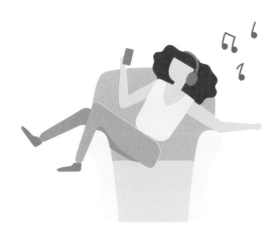

Keep the lights low

If you've tried lying in total darkness for a while and still can't get to sleep, perhaps you're still too wound up to properly switch off. Try creating a cosy atmosphere in your room with some dim lighting, and get yourself in the mood for relaxation. Make sure you don't turn on any lights that are too bright, though, as this will disrupt your sleep–wake cycle.

Meditate

After a long and tiring day, meditating can be a great way of clearing your head. If you find yourself feeling particularly anxious before bedtime, try the following meditation to help you feel more relaxed.

1. *Sit in a chair, keeping your back straight and your hands resting on your legs, or if you prefer to lie down, keep your arms relaxed at your sides.*

2. *Think about what is causing your anxiety and allow yourself to fully experience it.*

3. *Ask yourself why this thing, person or event is causing you so much anxiety. Do not make any judgement as to whether you think it's a worthy reason to feel upset or not.*

4. *Now start to think about your anxiety in the long-run. It is highly unlikely that the issues causing it are permanent. What can you do to improve things? Does it involve removing yourself from the situation, or having a chat to the person causing you distress?*

5. *Find comfort in the fact that you have acknowledged your anxiety and have gained a better understanding of it, enabling you to tackle it more effectively.*

Have a snack

It can be incredibly distracting if you feel hungry whilst you're trying to fall asleep. If you find yourself needing a quick pre-sleep snack, avoid anything heavy that could take too long to digest. Instead, go for some sleep-inducing foods that are high in potassium, such as bananas, avocado and pumpkin seeds.

Avoid alcohol

Whilst you may find that alcohol makes you feel
sleepier in the short-run, it can really impact the quality
of your sleep, leaving you feeling tired and groggy
the next morning. Try to resist the temptation of that
night cap and instead go for a chamomile tea or the
soothing drink on the next page.

Make a soothing drink

This delicious, creamy banana milkshake will help soothe and relax you. Bananas are great for helping you unwind, as they contain high levels of potassium which helps to keep your muscles relaxed.

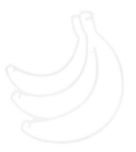

Soothing banana smoothie

250ml (8fl oz) milk or dairy-free alternative
1 banana, peeled and sliced
small handful of chopped dates
1 tablespoon honey for extra sweetness (optional)
pinch of cinnamon

Blend all the ingredients in a liquidizer or food
processor until smooth. You can even add a dollop of
plain yoghurt for extra creaminess, or try freezing your
bananas beforehand for a thicker, cooler drink in the
summer months.

Try not to have a lie-in tomorrow morning

This one might not be for tonight, but you'll need to know now as it'll help enormously with tomorrow evening.

When you can't get to sleep you may be seriously tempted to make up for any lost hours tomorrow morning, but this is only going to disrupt your sleep cycle further. Instead, try and get as much exposure to sunlight as you can tomorrow morning and keep caffeine intake to the first half of the day only.

Love and leave
your devices

If you find that you just can't resist looking at your
devices before you sleep, leave them downstairs
so you can't be tempted. If you rely on your phone
as an alarm, get yourself an alarm clock to do the
job instead.

Make sure your room is tidy

A clean and tidy room can make all the difference when you're trying to sleep. Declutter your room to declutter your mind.

Light a candle

Lighting a candle can create a cosy atmosphere in your room, helping you to relax and feel more at ease. Just remember to blow it out before going to sleep.

Wordsearch

Taking a few minutes out to do a simple puzzle like a
wordsearch can help distract yourself from any stress
and anxiety you may be experiencing, and will help you
to unwind at the end of a long day.

C	I	D	P	E	E	H	S	G	G	C	X	D	K	F
L	Z	N	K	X	E	T	A	T	I	D	E	M	H	K
T	R	R	O	G	B	N	Q	K	V	I	D	L	Z	M
B	D	B	G	O	N	I	D	I	E	D	Z	A	C	W
T	F	C	W	S	M	U	A	G	U	M	V	C	M	C
S	A	E	T	S	I	T	X	M	I	N	D	F	U	L
O	L	N	V	S	K	A	D	M	W	E	L	X	X	S
Z	H	H	H	V	L	G	G	G	U	E	I	H	C	X
A	T	I	P	E	N	I	V	S	J	O	L	E	E	P
B	N	W	R	I	Y	Z	Y	Z	Y	B	Y	R	I	C
E	R	B	N	Y	M	Y	U	C	G	G	R	B	N	W
B	L	E	N	T	G	I	J	P	N	E	U	A	F	Z
M	V	D	A	M	Q	O	B	J	K	I	V	L	G	C
E	D	T	K	T	Q	I	L	A	N	K	C	R	N	F
U	P	I	U	P	H	E	M	C	P	J	O	E	I	R
R	Z	M	E	G	V	I	Y	K	S	V	P	K	H	W
K	A	W	T	D	F	H	N	R	V	R	L	W	T	H
O	L	K	Z	E	J	X	Q	G	H	D	A	I	O	Z
S	J	J	G	U	I	R	W	O	C	H	K	T	O	A
Y	Z	O	G	R	V	H	M	H	D	W	U	Y	S	P

sleep	herbal	calm
stars	sheep	meditate
moon	breathing	mindful
sky	shine	soothing
bedtime	relax	evening

Don't worry

It's certainly easier said than done, but if you've been lying in bed wide awake for what feels like hours, try not to worry too much about it. You'll only work yourself up which will probably make things worse. Why not use the time to plan some relaxing, sleep-inducing things to do tomorrow evening?

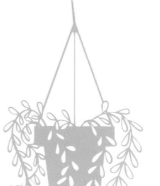

Get some plants
for your bedroom

Certain plants are great for purifying the air and can also help to improve sleep. Aloe Vera, English Ivy and Peace Lilies are especially good choices for your bedroom.

Listen

If you're having trouble relaxing before bedtime, try the following listening exercise to help ease your mind.

Find a comfortable position and close your eyes. Start to listen to your immediate surroundings. What sounds do you notice first? Now listen more closely. What smaller sounds can you hear? The quietest gurgle of a pipe perhaps, or a distant rumble of a car engine?

Make a list of all the things you can hear.

Would you rather

Who doesn't enjoy a classic game of would you rather? Decide on answers to the opposite to keep your brain distracted and occupied whenever you're feeling stressed or anxious.

Would you rather:

Be too cold or too warm

Be invisible or walk through walls

*Have to move to a new location every week
or stay in the place you were born forever*

Give up breakfast, lunch or dinner

*Be extremely overdressed or
underdressed for an occasion*

*Be stuck on an island by yourself or
with someone who never stops talking*

Don't clock-watch

It's never a good idea to look at the clock when you can't sleep, as you're only going to put more pressure on yourself. Turn around any clocks, and don't be tempted to check the time on your phone; ignorance is bliss.

Flush out any
excess caffeine

Regret having that late-night coffee or tea? If you're waiting for the caffeine-high to pass, drinking a glass of water can help to flush out any excess caffeine.

Find your pressure points

There are several pressure points on your body that, when 'activated', can help you relax. Try activating the following three points by gently applying pressure to them.

Hall of Impression Point: between your eyebrows

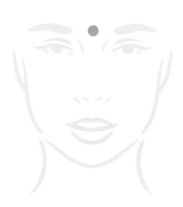

Heavenly Gate Point:
upper shell of the ear

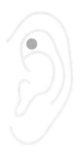

Inner Frontier Gate Point:
three fingers below the wrist

Fake it till you make it

Pretend to be really sleepy and you might just start to kid yourself into falling asleep. Imagine your eyelids feeling heavy and maybe even fake a yawn or two.

Fill deafening silence

Silence can be great for sleep, but do you ever get it
when the silence in your room is almost unbearable? If
so, then something as simple as opening the window
a crack to introduce a little bit of noise from outside
might help you relax.

Count backwards
from 100

As you count down, imagine yourself slowly drifting off.
Aim to completely relax the muscles in your arms and
legs by the time you reach zero.

100, 99, 98, 97, 96, 95, 94, 93, 92, 91, 90, 89, 88, 87, 86, 85, 84

Say the alphabet backwards

Harder than it sounds, but great for distracting your mind if you're having anxious or stressful thoughts. Take as long as you need the first time round, and then try and do it quicker.

Research something

Find out about something you've always been interested in to help distract you from any anxiety or tension you may be experiencing. Write down your favourite fact opposite and add to the list whenever you like.

Draw your emotions

Use the space below to draw how you're feeling right now. What colours would you choose and why?

Understanding how you're feeling will give you a better idea of how to right any wrongs.

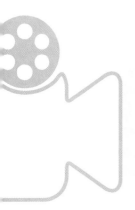

Have a
movie night

Fall asleep to your favourite film.
The comforting familiarity of the
words, music and sounds will
help you relax and feel calm in
your surroundings.

Stargaze

If it's a clear night, turn the lights off and have a peak out of your window at the stars. Take in the splendour of the night sky to help you relax and ease any tension in your body.

If it's a cloudy night, just take a look at the world outside, and notice how peaceful and quiet it is compared to daytime.

Count the sheep

It's the oldest trick in the book.

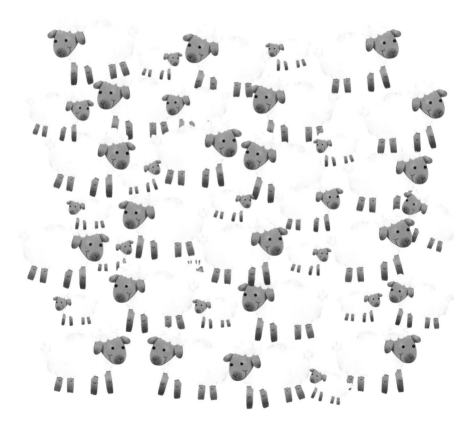

Make an easy herbal tea

Pop any of these herb combinations into a mug, pour over some hot water and enjoy. Each pairing will help cleanse and relax:

Lemongrass and ginger

Raspberry and mint

Fennel seed and orange

Go for a walk

If you're feeling particularly restless, it might be worth going for a quick walk round the block – or round the house if you don't feel like venturing outside – to try and burn any excess energy in your body.

Go to the toilet

Going to the toilet one more time before drifting off will lessen the chances of you needing to go in the middle of the night.

Dry your hair

If you've had a shower, make sure to dry your hair before getting into bed for maximum comfort. The last thing you need is a cold head and a wet pillow whilst you're trying to nod off.

Tie your hair back

If you have long hair, you might find it more comfortable to tie it back in a loose bun or ponytail.* This will keep it off your face so you don't have to worry about it disturbing you in the night.

*Use a loose hair tie or scrunchie to avoid damaging your locks.

Erase your fears

Using a pencil, do a rough sketch of some of your personal fears. Now rub it out, banishing them – and any other negative thoughts – from your mind as you do so.

Flip your mattress

If you never flip your mattress, you may find that it wears fairly quickly in some places. Try flipping it and see if the other side feels more comfortable.

You should aim to flip your mattress around every three months.

Only keep what's necessary

Take out any pillows or blankets you don't need for sleeping. They'll only get in the way or make the bed too hot as you're trying to drift off.

Invent something

Think up a new invention to distract yourself from any negative thoughts. Write down its name and what it does, then sketch what it looks like.

Draw yourself sleeping

What do you look like? What sleeping position are you in? Try to mimic what you've drawn and see if it makes you feel sleepier.

Get comfy

Make sure you're sleeping in something super comfortable. Keep it loose and light to make sure you don't get too hot as you sleep, and stick to breathable fabrics like cotton.

Take off jewellery

You may be used to jumping into bed without removing all of your jewellery. But taking those extra few seconds to do so – even any small ear studs – will probably help you feel much more comfortable and ready for bed.

Draw in response
to music

Put on some soft and gentle music, and use the
space below to draw whatever comes to mind to
distract yourself from not being able to sleep. Note how
the music affects your choice of colour and what
you decide to draw.

Mind map your thoughts

Map out your thoughts to get a better understanding of how you're feeling right now. Use the mini template below as a starting point, then create your own in the space opposite. What can you do to sort any negative feelings?

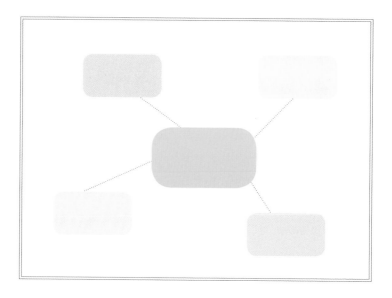

Organize something

Annoying pile of clothing in the corner of your room? Books all over the place? Organize something to declutter and clear your space, and, in turn, clear your mind.

Listen to an audiobook

Enjoy your favourite book with your eyes closed,
or pick a book with a narrator whose voice you
find particularly soothing.

Draw your best bits

Lift your mood and get rid of negative thoughts by using the space below to draw the things you like best about yourself, whether it's a physical attribute, a skill or an embodiment of your personality.

Cheat the sunset

It's always a good idea to expose your body to lots of light during the day. Then, when the light gradually fades in the evenings, your body understands that it's time for sleep. If you aren't able to do this, you can find alarm clocks that mimic the sunset by emitting bright light that slowly fades. They can also do the reverse, simulating sunrise in the mornings to help you wake up more naturally. There are plenty of these clocks available online.

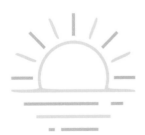

Keep water nearby

Do you ever wake up in the night really needing a drink? Keep some water on your bedside table so you don't end up having to get out of bed in the night.

Keep furry friends off the bed

It can be soothing to have your pet nearby as you sleep, but cats and dogs dream just like humans do and may move around in the night, disturbing your sleep and causing you to wake up. If it becomes a problem but you can't bring yourself to leave them downstairs, why not make a super comfy spot for them on the bedroom floor?

Keep the door closed

Sleeping with the door closed can create a sense of
security whilst you're trying to drift off, helping you to
feel calmer and more relaxed.

Get breakfast ready for the next day

Getting breakfast ready for the next day the night before will give you just that bit less to think about when you're trying to doze off.

List a few of your favourite breakfast ideas opposite to refer back to when needed.

Say goodnight

Saying goodnight to a loved one, and going to sleep on a happy and positive note, can make a huge difference. If you go to bed frustrated and in a bad mood, you will find it harder to switch off.

Don't go to bed in the middle of an argument

It is hugely important that you never go to bed in the middle of an argument. You will find that your quality of sleep is greatly affected by your negative state of mind.

Write a letter

If you have pent-up feelings about any unresolved arguments you've had with a loved one, and for whatever reason are unable to sort matters right now, write an apology note to them or a letter detailing your true feelings. You can choose whether or not you wish to send it to them the next morning, but for now it is important to get these thoughts out of your head so you can switch off for the night.

Dear _____

Ditch the duvet

Even in the cooler months, if your room is particularly warm it may be best to sleep with a blanket rather than a heavy duvet. Being too hot at night can affect the quality of your sleep.

Pamper yourself

Take the time to make yourself feel good before going to sleep. This could be anything from having a long bath to simply washing your face and making sure your skin feels clean before hitting the sack.

Think about the good things

Make a list of all the good bits from the past week.

....

....

....

....

....

....

....

....

....

....

...as well as the not-so-good

Make a list of the not-so-good bits. What can you do to overcome them?

Pack your bag

Packing your bag with everything you need for tomorrow will give you more time in the morning, and will give you one less thing to think about right now.

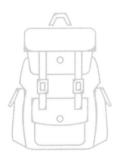

Decide what to wear

Deciding what to wear for the next day will also help clear your mind, leaving you feeling prepared and positive for the following morning.

Create a safe space

Making sure you feel safe and secure in your bedroom is extremely important and will help you relax when it comes to sleeping. How can you make your room feel that bit cosier? What do you need in your room to help you feel at ease?

Make a list of the top five items that help you feel safe and secure:

1...

....

2...

....

3...

....

4...

....

5...

....

Keep the floor clear

Keeping your bedroom floor clear of any items can be really helpful in case you need to get out of bed to go to the toilet in the middle of the night. If you know the floor is clear, then you won't need to turn on as many bright, sleep-interrupting lights.

Remove hanging items

Creepy shadow monster about to murder you in your sleep? Or just your dressing gown hanging on the back of your door? It might help to take down any hanging items for a distraction-free sleep.

Time with pets

You may have already read that it's best to keep your pets off of your bed, but if you're feeling stressed and anxious when trying to drift off, spending some time hanging out with your furry friend can make you feel better. Just make sure they don't follow you into bed when you're ready to sleep.

Try an oil burner

Electric oil burners are great for filling your room with soothing, sleep-inducing scents.

Scents to try:

Lavender
Vanilla
Bergamot
Sandalwood
Chamomile

Consider natural sleep aids

If you're having regular trouble getting off to sleep, you might want to consider sleep aids. You can get these over the counter. Chat to a pharmacist and see what they recommend.

Stop snoring

Snoring can be disruptive and affect your quality of sleep. Anti-snoring aids are also available over the counter.

What does your sleeping position say about you?

The positions we sleep in can tell us a lot about ourselves.

Stomach: *bold and social on the outside. Can be sensitive to criticism.*

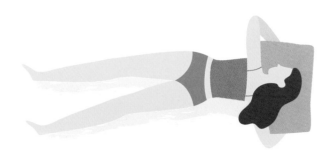

Back: *Can be quiet and reserved. Holds high standards for themselves.*

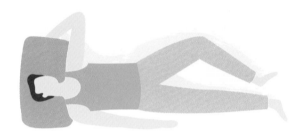

Side: *Can be shy at times, but relaxes and opens up after a short while.*

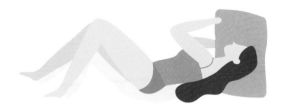

Stop working

Whatever you do, don't be tempted to catch up on missed emails or work-related tasks. Your bed is a place for sleep and relaxation, and you'll never be able to wind down if you're still thinking about work.

Imagine yourself sleeping

What do you look like and how does your body feel?
Does replicating these feelings now make you feel
sleepier?

Sleep in clean sheets

Making sure your bedding is clean can make you feel more comfortable at night time. What's better than the smell of fresh bed sheets anyway?

Keep essential items nearby

It's a good idea to keep anything you might need in the middle of the night nearby or at least in your room somewhere. That way you won't have to risk waking yourself up too much by having to get out of bed in search of a box of tissues or whatever else you might need.

Look through old photos

Revisiting old memories can be a great way to help you relax at bedtime.

Stick your favourite photo here, or write down your favourite memory for revisiting next time.

Lie still

Lie in bed completely still for as long as you can.
Starting with your feet and working your way up to your
head, imagine each part of your body slowly shutting
down for the night.

You do you

What are your own weird and wonderful sleep hacks?
Write them down here for next time.

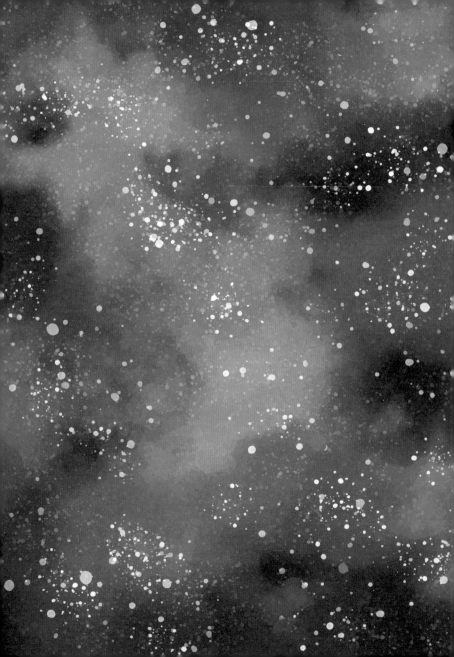